CHEMO EASE

Experiencing Chemotherapy Side Effects – How Natural Health Can Help

Lynda K Wilson-Hare

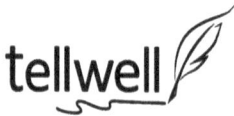

tellwell

Tellwell Talent
www.tellwell.ca

ISBN
978-0-2288-5619-1 (Hardcover)
978-0-2288-5609-2 (Paperback)
978-0-2288-5620-7 (eBook)

Foreword

The purpose of this book is to try and help people who are afflicted with cancer and those who have the difficult job of caregiver or support provider as they watch a loved one go through an extremely difficult time.

I do not write this book to talk about cures or to talk about recovery. These are miracles that few will witness. I write this book to help reduce the suffering and uncomfortable sensations that result when a person has chemotherapy. The book is realistic. I hope not to set up anyone for failure, but to try to give options to provide ease and maintain quality of life for as long as you have.

I have spent years studying traditional natural medicine, and I have researched many studies on its effectiveness. I do not spend much time on all of the 'ins and outs' of these research journals and documents, but I do reference them should you want to know the nitty-gritty. My intention in this book is to try and find natural herbs that could relieve the chemotherapy side effects. I apply my knowledge and what I found in my journey to help others hold on to a quality of life during treatment. This is not a fact-finding research study but a guide of simple, obtainable things that can help you or your loved one.

I have set this book up into two parts. You can choose to read the story, my thoughts, and some research on our journey. Or, if you prefer to go to the section on herbs/problem-solving, I have a table of contents to help guide you. You can also use the table of contents for future reference.

—

Disclaimer

While all care is taken with the accuracy of the facts and procedures in this book, the author accepts neither liability nor responsibility to any person with respect to loss, injury, or damage caused or alleged to be caused directly or indirectly by the information contained in this book. The purpose of this book is to educate and inform. For medical advice, you should seek the personal advice and services of your health care professional. Material provided as research from scientific and medical publications has been selected according to the author's personal criteria. Any oversight is unintentional. It is also important to point out that some supplements can interfere with or reduce the effectiveness of the performance of certain medications. Therefore, before taking any supplements, it is critical that you speak with your doctor to ensure your health will not be adversely affected.

Dedications

For my darling Husband Bruce,

I am so blessed to share my life with you. Thanks for believing in me, inspiring me, and encouraging me. You have been my rock, and you have been there every step of the way for me. Your faith in me has been incredible; your strength and passion in supporting this path have made the biggest obstacles seem surmountable. You never questioned anything I gave you; you just believed. Thank you for this incredible journey that never would have happened without your influence, your motivation, and, most importantly, your love.

For my Mom Hilda,

Although you have long passed, your positive influence, making time for others, and example to live life to the fullest still resonate with me. Your courage, strength, wisdom, and humour will inspire me always. I am also eternally grateful for a childhood of bare feet, country walks, exploring nature, and loving and caring for animals.

Table of Contents

Why Write this Book?

You may wonder why, as a traditional natural health practitioner, I am endorsing chemotherapy. Well, until you have been confronted with a life-threatening disease, please do not pass judgement on others who are trying to find their way of extending life. As terrible as chemotherapy is, it has been prolonging life for cancer victims for years now – and this is incredible, given that 10 years ago the extension was only months. My goal is not to question the path you choose, but to provide you with options to problem-solve finding relief for some of the side effects by using natural sources. Chemotherapy has been around since 1940 and is still the main treatment recognized by the medical profession for cancer management.

Typically, when side effects start, a potpourri of other medications are given to you to take as needed. Hence, it gets really difficult to determine what is causing the side effect and why you feel horrible. Fewer medications, less side effects and complications is our goal in having the chemotherapy work to the fullest extent. Symptoms arise as the body's best efforts to heal itself. We do not want to suppress the body's natural response and inhibit the healing process, but we do need to make this process be less uncomfortable.

Let's never forget that chemotherapy is extremely dangerous – just look at all the personal protective equipment (gloves, gowns, and masks) your nurse must wear to give you your treatment.

Chemotherapy drugs are outright poisons, classed as biohazard where even excretions are toxic waste. Spilling it on your skin will cause a major burn. Chemo kills cancer cells; however, it cannot tell the difference between healthy cells. In particular chemo has a direct effect on the bone marrow. Bone marrow develops white blood cells that are responsible for our immune system. With limited production of these cells the patient becomes unable to fight infection. Red blood cells, and platelet production are also affected. Simply put, red blood cells bring nutrients and oxygen to the cells, and platelets are essential for blood clotting. All having major impact on number and size of blood cell production and how quickly the body regenerates while on chemotherapy treatment.

For those of you who are against chemotherapy, I would like to point out a very positive side effect that you may not be aware of. The process of going to get treatment while sitting and talking with people who are going through similar issues provides very good mental health support. You can think of it as a strange social club. I have had the luxury of seeing cancer clinics where they promote a social club environment that really makes the patients look forward to it.

Once someone is sick, there is a tendency to not visit or call as there is fear that they will not be feeling well, or that visitors may bring a virus/bacterium to an immunocompromised person. Far worse is the person who is afraid to see the individual who is sick out of fear that they will look sickly and the visitor won't know how to react. What happens is the person who is not feeling well and who is unable to do their regular life routine will now feel abandoned. Sometimes the person feels so terrible that they do not want anyone to visit. At least the treatment visits help fill some of this void by ensuring communal gatherings with people who understand what they are going through and how they are feeling.

Two situations in my life have caused me to see that quality of life is the most important aspect of health. My mother was diagnosed with cancer in the bowel that moved to the liver. Her suffering was horrible. I had just started my Natural Health Ph.D. and I felt absolutely powerless in trying to help her. Symptoms that she was experiencing did not make sense medically to me. Herbs that would work in a healthy person did not have the same result for my mother when she was on chemotherapy. I have come to realize that when a person is on medication – any meds, not just chemo – the side effects that show as symptoms do not respond to herbs in the same way that a healthy, non-medicated person would. While trying to find positive improvements with my mother's health, we monitored closely any changes. This ended up being very heart-breaking as she deteriorated so quickly.

Many years later, my husband developed cancer in the bowel that has manifested in the liver. This time, I was ready to figure out a plan of attack for how we were going to fight this cancer off and work on a cure. But life has a funny way of setting you back and saying start again. Remembering not to set markers for improvement, we started slowly. We sought to improve any symptoms that arose while building an arsenal of herbs so that the side effect medication rebounds would not add to him feeling horrible. We focused on quality and on how to get him feeling good and able to do the important things in life. It was also important to focus on what was important to him. For example, I had not realized how important a full head of hair was to him. Be aware of these things – we may not think they are big in the overall scheme of things, but what is important to that person is what you need to focus on. For them it means they regain their quality of life. The more chemotherapy they take, the more side effects begin to accumulate and adapt, hence taking on different or more intense side effects. The way the body releases the chemo toxin from your body changes depending on the length of time you are on it.

I am providing you with options. Pick what is important to you/your loved one and start there. Don't try to do everything at once. Take small steps. Know that as the body adapts to the treatment, these small victories may not work as effectively and you may need a new approach. This is why I am offering a few varieties.

Needless to say, I understand the extreme discomfort and helplessness that a person on chemo is having. I believe my mission is to try and help you find small pieces of relief that will provide you with some hope/quality of life.

I add this quotation to help us see the importance of having a quality of life so that we can experience joy:

> Yes, we suffer pain, we become ill, we die. But we also hope, laugh, celebrate, we know the joy of caring for one another, often we are healed and we recover by many means. We do not have to pursue the flattening out of human experience. I invite all to shift their gaze, their thoughts, from worrying about health care to cultivating the art of living. And, today with equal importance, the art of suffering, the art of dying.
>
> (Illich I., 1994, p4)
> PRINTED WITH PERMISSION

What You Need to Know

Firstly – be informed. Be curious about your situation, track your symptoms, and ask your oncology doctor or nurses questions. Keep a journal; do not rely on memory. Keeping a record will allow you to see trends and remember what worked or what didn't work should the scenario present itself again. You don't need to keep a daily record, just when something happens. I suggest you keep this record handy. Post it on the refrigerator, for example, so that it is convenient to write in. Find out as much as you can about your situation. Listen to the health professionals but think the problem through for yourself and make your own judgements and decisions. Maintaining your independence is key. If you do not understand, it is your right to be given an explanation. Do not feel shy or uncomfortable. Know that health professionals talk about body functions all the time; do not be embarrassed. Make your doctor your partner. It is also very difficult to judge between trustworthy information and 'quackery.' The question of who and what to believe is a very important one to you. The best advice is to approach all recommendations for health and well-being with a lot of skepticism. Consider all sides of an issue, including the credibility of the speaker before coming to a conclusion. Investigate, look at recommendations, and see if there is a 'buyer beware' controversy. Truth is not in mass or social media. Take responsibility in the form of reading, thinking, making decisions, and asking. Don't let your life be determined by influences of mass media.

As a traditional natural health practitioner, I can attest to this sad situation. I have witnessed clerks in health food stores offer miracle cures without any formal education or consideration to what the person's diagnosis may be or what other medications they may be on. Reading on the internet or watching an infomercial does not make you an expert – buyer beware.

Secondly, change your mindset. I think that in many cases we set ourselves up for failure when we talk about the fight against cancer. We know that the profitability of pharmaceutical companies is in long-term pharmaceutically-managed medical conditions, not in cures. All you have to do is ask people what medications they are taking. It is a rare situation to find anyone over the age of 50 who is not on some form of medication. In 2020, 75% of all television commercials were advertisements for drugs and the five biggest pharma companies declared they spent more on marketing than on research (Snyder, 2021).

What I propose is much easier to handle. Following each visit to the oncologist with my mother, we would problem-solve next steps of how she would know she was getting better. Each time it became more and more upsetting until we stopped talking about it. The best approach is not to look at cancer going away (being cured). We know that cancer can return even after five years of remission (Canadian Cancer Society, 2021). So, it is really important to not keep tabs. Look forward to the cancer as a stable disease while **focusing on no growth**. If you have shrinkage, be happy, but know that cancer cells stay in your system for a long time. They can adapt and begin growth again. Don't despair; it is the body's natural defence to adapt. Focusing on growth and constant changes creates more stress which enhances the environment for cancer to thrive.

Our bodies are always exposed to viruses, bacteria, hazardous products and even cancer cells on a frequency basis that we are not even aware of. Our immune system responds to these threats so efficiently that we do not even realize our health was at risk.

It is really important that you do not dwell on what caused the cancer. In some cases, people have had direct exposures and are aware of what caused their disease. I am referring more to the people who have no idea why they were chosen. There are many reasons why a person could get cancer and the options are endless. I tend to think that in many cases the reason is chronic unresolved stress.

Excessive stress wreaks havoc on our immune systems.

People who get themselves into situations where they are powerless to find a way out experience long periods of ongoing stress. Our bodies are designed with the 'fight or flight' system, and so when we are exposed to stress, we have options to save ourselves. As time evolves, our ability to stand our ground and fight are limited, and the ability to run away is even less of an option. Stress causes the hormone cortisol to be released which in turn causes our adrenal glands to produce adrenaline to give us the boost to fight on or run away. Our adrenal glands are forced to work constantly to maintain our prolonged high-alert state. With no rest, the adrenal gland becomes imbalanced. High cortisol can be the trigger for adrenal stress symptoms and related long-term health problems such as chronic fatigue, lack of energy, sleep disruption, depression, increased cravings, and weakened immunity. Our bodies can exist in one of two states: 1) growth, repair, and rebuilding mode; or 2) protection mode. The longer the body remains in protection mode (high alert), there is no energy applied to renewal and regrowth. This redirection of energy makes a lot of sense when we are facing a bear – in moments of life versus imminent death, digestion, and reproduction become much less important. But what happens when the bear is long gone yet the high stress response lingers? The only way to decrease the production of cortisol is to get out of the protection mode – triggered by quick breathing, increased heart rate. This means relaxing. Yes, take a stressed person and tell them to relax, doesn't work so well. Deep breathing and meditation work, but only if you can change your mindset to get into this state. Walking in nature has proven very helpful where the rich oxygen environment from trees and plants help to unconsciously breathe deeply – the old saying take; time to smell the flowers. Another hint, emotional distressed – sit down and have a good cry – let it all out. During times like this, tears will release cortisol, which in turn resets the body to repair mode. It is truly helpful to let the tears flow. Stress shuts down our metabolism so we cannot get proper nutrition, and with added cravings we reach for food that is not healthy causing our bodies to go into a state of acidosis and low oxygen levels As I explain later, cancer cannot exist or grow in an oxygen-rich or slightly alkaline environment.

Cancer, as with any life-threatening disease, makes us stop and rethink our lives and choices. Have we done all we wanted? Do we have regrets? What do we want to let go of? For the person with cancer, this in itself can help to reframe (change your mindset) and focus on what is important. What do you want out of the rest of your life? Resetting expectations and determining quality of life are essential to getting in the right perspective for living with a stable disease, stopping the cycle of chronic stress, and living the life that is important to you. It is your 'new normal' – get comfortable with it. I am in no way saying pack up your stuff and make your will. I am saying discard what is making you uncomfortable and look after you. This book is not a mental health/stress-relieving self-help book; there are plenty of those on the market. Better yet, there are many wonderful, qualified professionals out there to talk to and help you either understand the source of your stress or provide support on how to manage your situation.

Going through chemotherapy is very difficult – think of it as poison in your system injected directly into your bloodstream. Drink lots of water, even though you don't feel like it, to flush it out. As soon as it is diluted, you will start to feel better. The chemo leaves your body by many routes – bladder, bowels, saliva, and sweat. So be prepared to have symptoms anywhere.

Remember I mentioned how quickly cancer can adapt, so that the way you feel after one treatment can be very different to the next? Don't be alarmed – anticipate it. Most importantly, for two or three days after chemo do not stress your body. Drink lots of water, take supplements, and rest. You will complain about being tired and feeling awful, but the more you rest in those few days, the faster your blood will rebuild and you will start to feel better and be able to do some quality living at the level of your new norm. So many times, I had to reinforce this with my husband as feeling tired and awful is so hard to see past. Over these two or three days, focus on reading, puzzles, movies, and computer games so that if you fall asleep, it's no big deal. Think about your blood building back up so that your body can get the energy it needs.

All life is adaptable and resilient. This is the ability to bounce back, and to adapt to new ways of thinking, feeling and acting. One of the key messages for anyone experiencing cancer is to learn to let go of things outside of your control. Letting go means allowing yourself to stop unproductive worrying while shifting your attention to activities where you can make a difference or participate in positively. Identify behaviours that might come from worry or fear such as doing everything yourself, withdrawing from others, or being curt with family/co-workers. Do it differently tomorrow.

What is Cancer, and How Does this All Work?

Never forget that cancer is your body, your cells, not a foreign intruder. It is your body's desperate attempt for self preservation when all other mechanisms have failed. Cancer cells are normal, healthy cells that have genetically mutated and are capable of living without oxygen. In an amazing part of our natural makeup, these cells somehow are encouraged to start growing faster than normal. In fact, minimal differences between healthy and cancerous cells. When our immune system is compromised, it allows an opening for cancer to develop. There are not enough white blood cells to attack the damaged cells and remove the dead ones. Newly created cells take on the mutated form and accumulate to form tumors. Cancer treats our healthy cells as a host, pulling away the good nutrients and blood so our bodies waste. The cancer is very smart and very adaptive, even creating its own blood supply. It can take poisons like chemotherapy and radiation and not only adapt but in some cases continue to grow.

Let's face it: cancer is our reality. It is the leading cause of death according to the World Health Organization. Almost one in two people in the population will now develop cancer at some time in their life. This is 45% of men and 43% of women (Canadian Cancer Society, 2021).

Key factors to be aware of Yeast (Candida)

Candida coexists with cancer and acts as a glue to keep the cancer cells together. The fungus produces an acid. Candida plays a vital role in the cancer's ability to survive by making toxins and allowing mutated cells to replicate into full-blown cancer. As yeast grows out of control, it can manifest as symptoms such as gas, bloating, constipation, depression, fatigue, and brain fog. During chemotherapy, candida festers due to the weakened immune system, showing toxicity. As a result, candida is seen on the surface of the tongue. This is known as thrush.

Sugar – especially refined

Cancer cells gather their energy to multiply from carbohydrates, it is easier since this metabolising process does not require oxygen. Do not ingest corn syrup or refined white sugar. Sugar can lead to fermentation in the body that feeds and promotes yeast growth and bad bacteria, suppressing the immune system. White sugar is harmful because it has been stripped of all its vital nutrients. In addition, artificial sweeteners and aspartame are not only toxic and addictive, but they also have a high glycaemic index. This means that upon being ingested, they raise blood sugar levels very quickly. This causes the body to use more insulin, so it stores fat faster, creating weight gain. So, although the sweetener has zero calories, this process actually causes you to gain weight – again, buyer beware!

A sweet alternative is stevia. South Americans have used stevia for centuries to sweeten. Stevia can be used liberally as it has the least effect on blood sugars and has zero effect on glycaemic index. Note – look at the ingredients to ensure that there have been no mixtures (fillers) with the stevia such as aspartame or you will not get what you want. Raw honey, and maple syrup are natural sugars that still contain vitamins and minerals.

Antioxidants: Nature's sponges

Very important to note is antioxidants, or free radical scavengers. They are the body's method of neutralizing nasty particles. Basically, these are little sponges that soak up harmful chemicals. The most important ones are vitamin E and C which I provide more information on later. The brain normally has the highest concentrations of vitamin C in the body. The advantage of these antioxidants is that they can easily enter the blood brain barrier and reach the brain cells where they are needed most.

The blood brain barrier is believed to exist in the capillaries within the brain where it is capable of keeping harmful compounds from getting into it. If the level of antioxidants is reduced in the body, then the brain can no longer protect itself and the chemicals cross into the brain cells. For example, after an injury to the brain or nervous system, our body metabolism speeds up. This generates more free radicals. The brain uses the antioxidants quickly and depletes the source unless extra doses of vitamin C, E, or other antioxidants are taken.

Herbal guidance

So now you know why I was passionate to write this book. Let's move on to what wonderful sources Mother Nature has provided us with that can help make this process more bearable.

There are many wonderful herbs to choose from. The list I am providing is comprised of specimens that I have used which have demonstrated the effect I wanted to achieve. I am not discounting that other herbs could do something similar or maybe better, but at the time of writing this book, these are the herbs I know will work and are easy to obtain.

I have divided this chapter into three sections:

❖ Essential herbs
❖ Nutritional herbs, substances, and vitamins
❖ Other natural information

It is often very hard to swallow tablets or capsules either due to the effects of chemotherapy; feeling nauseated, or even low energy. The positioning of the cancer can also make swallowing painful. The good news is that many herbs now come in a liquid form. These tinctures can be added to water for drinking rather than swallowing tablets or capsules.

Drugs are excreted from the body from the organs -kidneys, liver, skin, and lungs. We also eliminate drugs from the body by feces, urine, mucus, saliva and tears. As such, in looking at your potential side effects, these herbs will focus on protecting the tissue or getting rid of the hazardous waste from that area. As chemotherapy is excreted/expelled, you may develop burning or itching sensations – like bugs crawling – or sores as the 'poison' is pushed from the body.

❖ Essential herbs

These typically do not interfere with your chemotherapy or medication regime (although I do recommend you discuss these with your physician before taking). These herbs are used to help restore, tone, and invigorate systems in the body to promote general health and well-being. Below, I describe how these herbs support the body.

Marigold

This hidden gem has incredible healing power. Yes, this is regular old marigold which you can buy in garden centres anywhere. It is a low maintenance plant that is easy to grow. I usually plant about four of them in my garden and they provide enough flower petals to last for the year.

Marigold has wound-healing properties. It is antiseptic, antifungal, and antibacterial to promote healing. It has a fantastic ability to heal herpes-type viruses, specifically cold sores and cankers – inflamed or ulcerated conditions. We have found it incredible for giving relief and healing to sores in the mouth and skin caused by chemotherapy. The antifungal properties make it effective on thrush (candida). It is also useful as a digestive remedy because it stimulates the flow of bile.

Here is how you harvest the marigold, but also know that if you have no ability to grow the plant or it is the wrong season, you can buy it in teabag form (see section titled "Where can I buy these herbs and vitamins?").

Use the dried bloom – you can either leave it on the stem until it dries or cut the bloom once it has lost its full prime and then let it dry in the sunshine. Remove the bloom from the stem. The petals have the healing properties.

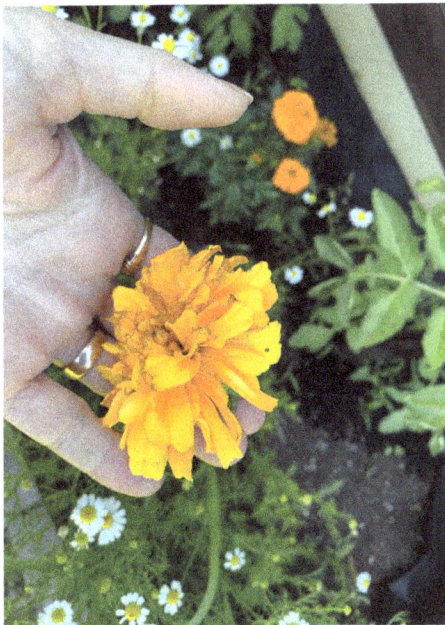

Marigold flower

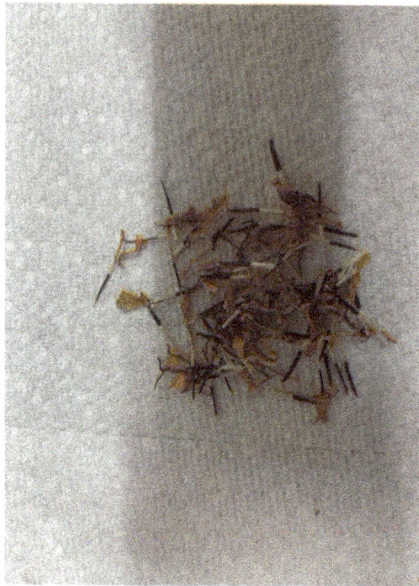

Marigold petals

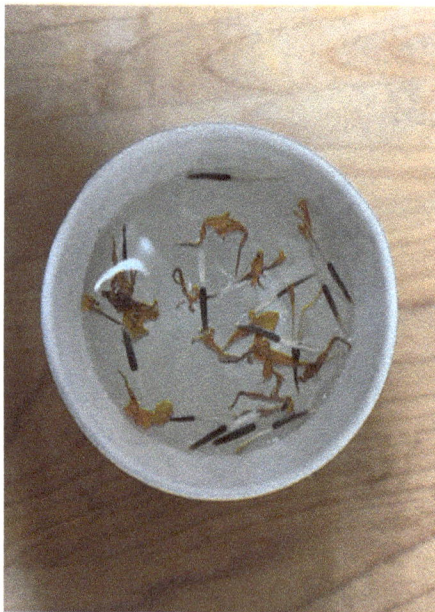

Marigold brew

To brew – I soak a pinch of the petals in one cup of hot water (not boiled) overnight, like steeping tea. I remove the petals in the morning. When I am using the mixture frequently, I make enough for a couple of days in a sealed (preferably glass) container. Since there is no preservative (note that alcohol is not good for liver), it is only good for a short time.

How to use:

For sores in the mouth – Take as soon as you feel irritation. Gargle and do not rinse out your mouth after. You can swallow the mixture as well. There is no problem with swallowing the mixture as it is also good for digestion. I also know that the sores in the mouth may work their way down the esophagus, so swallowing the marigold brew will help heal those sores. Take the Marigold rinse as soon as you notice the sores. The longer you wait, more sores will develop and it will take longer and be more difficult to heal them.

Cold sores (sores on lip) – Mix the marigold with your favourite lip balm or use in a chemical-free cream and apply it.

Sores on skin – You can use the marigold tea as a wash. Apply the liquid to a cotton pad and dab over the skin where the sores are. These sores can also appear on the scalp under your hair. Here, you can use the tea as a rinse if there are multiple sores to get at. Dab or pour the marigold brew on your scalp and let it dry. Since it is water-based, it will not make your hair oily.

You can also take a mild cream (no fragrances or chemicals) and mix in some of the concentrated marigold tea. When you put the cream on your skin, the marigold will be absorbed with the cream. The cream also keeps the marigold on the skin for a longer period, while the water-based wash will evaporate as well as absorb. Sometimes the sores are really tender, so spraying or dabbing the wash will cause less discomfort than applying the cream.

Astragalus

One of my favourite herbs, Astragalus is known as a tonic. A tonic has the ability to increase the body's resistance to stress. This means that it takes a lot more stress to move a person off-centre when they are using tonics on a daily basis. These herbs are defined as substances that are provided by nature for the repair and maintenance of normal physiology. They do not stress the body but are suitable for long-term use. Tonics differ from most medicinal substances in being bidirectional so if the herb senses lacking – it supports. However, if the herb senses an abundance, it reduces concentration. Hence correcting the illness or imbalance, it is truly miraculous.

Chinese herbalists have recommended Astragalus to help the body build up energy and resist diseases and infections. Conventional medical researchers expressed interest in the possibility that Astragalus might boost immune response and lessen the side effects of chemotherapy.

I attribute the use of Astragalus in my husband's treatment for him not losing his sense of taste or appetite while on chemotherapy. Although we were told that a change or complete loss of taste would happen over time, after three years it never occurred. This very positive attribute of Astragalus helped to ensure he kept eating and more importantly enjoying food.

During my Ph.D. thesis, I used Astragalus as the medium to see the effect it had on my test group for reducing stress. The response was incredible (Wilson-Hare, 2007).

Milk Thistle

The liver is one of the busiest organs in the body, working constantly to breakdown food for blood transport and metabolize waste for excretion through urine or feces. Since the liver does all this processing, it is the most exposed organ to hazardous chemicals such as chemotherapy.

Milk thistle's active ingredient is silymarin, and silymarin is capable of regenerating damaged liver cells and protecting against injury due to alcohol, hepatitis, and industrial liver toxins. Milk thistle is also used medically to treat chronic inflammatory liver conditions. (Ottoboni & Ottoboni, 2004). In addition to being one of the best-known liver protectors, it reduces liver congestion and prevents toxins from penetrating the liver cells. Milk thistle contains large amounts of extraordinarily therapeutic substances known as flavonoids. Milk thistle is known to protect and heal the liver in three primary ways:

- It acts directly on the cell membranes of the liver by stabilizing and strengthening structure. This reduces the ability of toxins to bind to the receptor sites that milk thistle is attracted to. This allows liver cells to regenerate.
- Toxins are cycled continuously between the gastrointestinal tract and the liver, thereby increasing the ability to cause more damage with each pass. Milk thistle interrupts the primary absorption of toxins preventing reabsorption with further enterohepatic circulation.
- It stimulates protein synthesis (Mowrey, 1993).

Even if the cancer has not affected the liver, it is important to ensure that this special organ gets all the nutrients to help maintain its health and functions during chemo.

Burdock

Burdock clears lymph and liver congestion. It has antimicrobial activity to help clean the blood. Burdock has the ability to heal skin conditions and build a healthy immune system. Burdock appears to slow the growth of tumours (Fitzgerald, 2001).

Red clover

Red clover promotes cleansing of the blood through antiseptic and antibiotic actions. It supports the elimination of toxin in the urine. It has an anti-cancer compound called genistein (Fitzgerald, 2001).

Ginkgo biloba

As chemotherapy starts to accumulate in the body, it enters the blood brain barrier and causes 'chemo brain.' Poor memory, depression, anxiety, brain fog, and numbness are all part of nervous system toxicity, and ginkgo helps to reduce this.

Horsetail

Horsetail is a primary source of silicon. It is necessary for growth and repair of bone and tissue. Horsetail stimulates many cellular metabolic processes that are the basis for the repair of connective tissue and bone. For chemotherapy patients, horsetail is essential in the formation of osteoblasts – bone-forming cells – that make up our blood (Mowrey, 1993). Horsetail helps stimulate the circulation in the scalp, and the silica gives the hair body. During chemotherapy, hair thins or falls out. Using horsetail helps to regenerate the tiny blood vessels in the scalp to reduce the amount of hair falling out. You can take this orally, or you can put the herb in warm water and massage into the scalp. Although my husband's hair thinned when he first started chemo, I believe the horsetail supplements were the reason he did not lose it all or even clumps. He was also able to regrow any loss quickly.

Aloe vera

Aloe Vera gel is naturally rich in antioxidants, including vitamins C, E, and A. It also provides a naturally cooling sensation when applied. As such it provides relief for sunburn, redness, itchiness and cuts.

As the chemotherapy excretes out of the skin, sometimes we found that we had to change from marigold to aloe to find relief. Aloe gel is thicker and can be easier to work with in some areas. For example, burning sensation around the anus due to diarrhea can be relieved with aloe vera gel.

Aloe vera juice also has medicinal benefits, but with no preservatives it must be used quickly. If ingested, the juice can help ease stomach issues.

Lemon balm (Melissa officinalis): Reducing body's response to stress naturally

Lemon balm has amazing soothing properties to disperse depression. It is a perennial, it is easy to grow, and it spreads quickly. It can be purchased at any garden centre. You use the fresh leaves, picked before the plant flowers.

The great physician Avicenna recommended this plant because it makes the heart *merry*. The herb is recommended for nervousness, depression, insomnia, and nervous headaches. It is antimicrobial, antiviral, antispasmodic, and antihistamine. So, in addition to reducing the physical effects associated with stress, lemon balm also helps sooth an upset stomach – all essential characteristics to calm the effects of chemotherapy. I have witnessed people that were fretful and anxious, and upon drinking one cup of lemon balm tea, watch that tension fall away from their face.

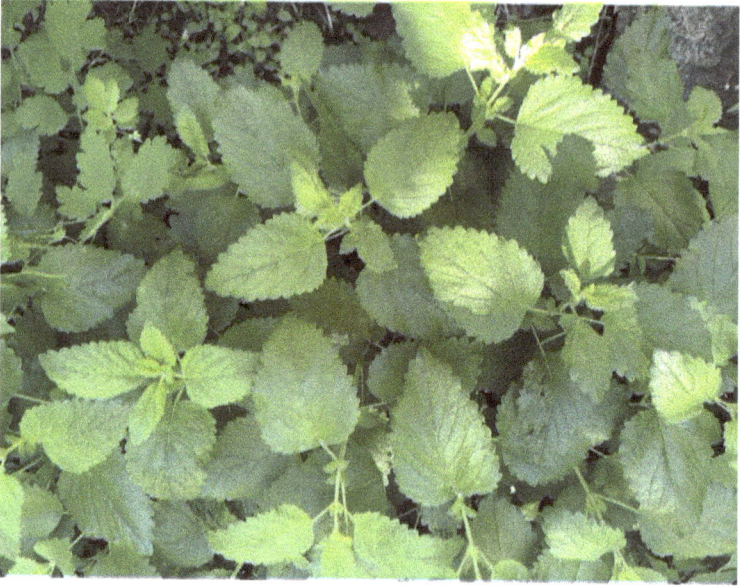

Lemon Balm

How to brew – Take leaf and make small tears in it. It has a lovely lemon smell. Take a cup of hot water and put the leaf in the cup, like brewing tea. When the drink is ready, the leaf will sink to the bottom of the cup. There is no need to remove it. The tea has a flavour of green tea with lemon. It is tasty, and without realizing it, you will find your tension has reduced. I will add the fresh leaf to other teas as well with the same effect. On hot summer days, I put the leaves in ice water. Again, when it sinks you can enjoy the mild taste with the same effect.

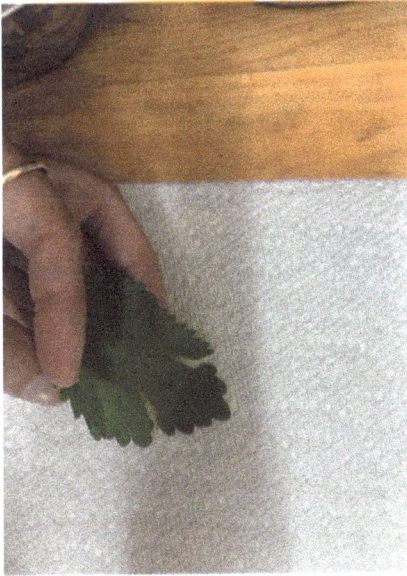

Lemon Balm Leaf

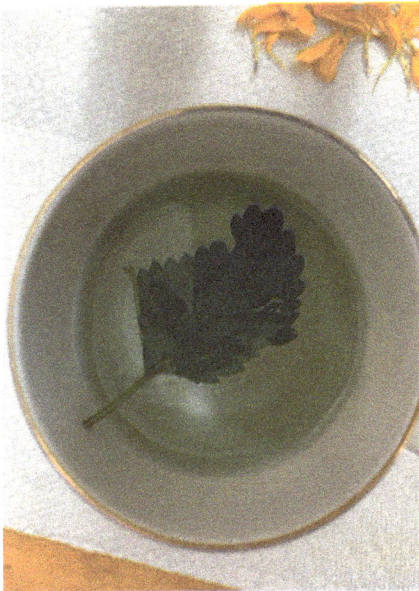

Lemon Balm Brew

The leaf is best freshly cut, but can be dried, however it does lose some of its properties. In preparation for winter, I pick the leaves, wash them, and freeze them.

Other ways to relax are to add a few lemon balm leaves with small tears to your bath water, or use the leaves in a compress to relax your eyes.

❖ Nutritional herbs, substances, and vitamins

Nutritional herbs

Our bodies require many vitamins, minerals, amino acids and enzymes to process so that your cells can use it. Pharmaceuticals can cause problems in the body's ability to digest any or all of these nutrients. In turn, drugs, stress, alcohol, the nutrients listed all have the ability to increase or decrease how the pharmaceutical performs. This is very important. My husband was a type 2 diabetic for 30+ years. When he started on chemotherapy, his blood sugars dropped dangerously low and extremely fast at night. He had never had this history and it was very scary for both of us. It took a long time to regulate. Fortunately, we were able to utilize herbs and refrain from medication; however, this is another story.

Drugs have a profound effect on how the body handles nutrients. They can cause some nutrients to be excrete in higher than normal quantities. If the drugs are causing these nutrients to be washed out of the body, then your cells will be lacking these essential elements. Absorption of nutrients becomes less efficient and the nutrient requirement may change, with some diminishing and some increasing. When you are on chemotherapy, your daily living schedule will change. Less physical activity and a reduced appetite may result in small, more frequent meals, maybe even more fast food (poorer quality food) which will create loss of energy (Ottoboni & Ottoboni, 2002).

Many cancer patients die not of cancer but of starvation as a result of a much diminished appetite or impaired digestive function or both. If other aspects of a cancer patient's health are optimized, they should logically be able to mount a better resistance (Vanderlinden & Vucenik, 2004). Cancer itself can cause nutritional deficiencies and so can the medications used to treat it. Both cancer and chemotherapy can cause loss of appetite, nausea, intestinal absorption problems, and increased metabolism (calorie burning), all of which can lead to malnourishment and weight loss (Frei, Quillin, & Bloomfield, 1996).

It is important to note, nutrition should not be used as a sole therapy for cancer treatment. However, nutrition can dramatically improve the quantity and quality of life and the chances for remission. (Frei, Quillin, & Bloomfield, 1996).

When taking chemotherapy, it is natural not to feel like eating. The problem with not eating is that all your energy is then collected by the cancer cells or excreted as waste without the normal cells getting the goodness. It is very important that your healthy cells get nourishment so that they can generate new blood cells and you can begin to feel more energy. This is where the nutritional capsules come in. Even if you can eat, sometimes it is difficult to get all the nutrition that you need. When my husband was having good days, I still ensured that he took these three nutrients which can be found in capsules, tablets, or in a powder supplement.

Desiccated liver

Desiccated beef liver supplements are beef liver that has been dried, ground into powder, and capsulized. The liver is where the body stores many vitamins and minerals, so beef liver is naturally rich in vitamin A, vitamin B12, copper, folate, riboflavin, hyaluronic acid, and many other nutrients. These capsules also contain eight out of the nine essential amino acids, making it beneficial for tissue repair and protein synthesis.

Spirulina

Spirulina is a potent source of nutrients. It contains a powerful plant-based protein called phycocyanin. Research shows this may have antioxidant, pain-relieving, anti-inflammatory, and brain-protective properties.

Spirulina also contains protein; vitamins B1, B2, and B3; copper; iron; magnesium, potassium, and manganese; and small amounts of almost every other nutrient that you need.

Vitamin C combined with spirulina prevents elevated levels of liver enzymes (ALT and AST), a signal of cell death. Note that chemotherapy greatly affects both these levels. You can see your results in blood work.

Barley grass

Barley grass has impressive antioxidant content; along with vitamin C, vitamin E, and beta-carotene, barley grass is a potent supplier of the critical enzyme superoxide dismutase which helps neutralize the effects of oxygen free radicals. Barley grass helps to repair blood vessels and bone marrow.

Barley grass has the ability to stimulate gut-friendly bacteria. It has been found to assist in alleviating inflammation in the bowel by absorbing toxins accumulating there. With chemotherapy, the onset of diarrhea may be curbed with taking barley grass. I suggest that it be taken daily, and add extra when diarrhea starts. However, we have found that for the first two to three days of chemotherapy, although barley grass is taken, because of the rapid onset of diarrhea, it is necessary to take a pharmaceutical if it does not stop within an hour. Again it is about quality of life, and not spending your day on the toilet. Also you do not want to become dehydrated and lose precious nutrients.

Essential vitamins

There is a great deal of material out there to explain why eating well still means you need to take vitamins (for the healthy person) but here is a quick summary:

- Soil the food is grown in is depleted of essential minerals;
- Time from farmer to table is weeks, and by then important vitamins have been depleted (e.g. vitamin C).
- Our bodies are assaulted with environmental pollutants and stress; therefore, we need to boost our immune system.
- Very few people actually eat a balanced diet.

In one supplement, you can get a daily intake of 1,000 mg of Vitamin C – or drink eight glasses of fresh squeezed orange juice (Mindell & Hopkins, 2003).

Vitamin D

Vitamin D comes naturally from sunshine exposure. In the supplement vitamin D3, the 3 refers to the mix of plant and animal ingredients that hosts the strongest form of Vitamin D (cholecalciferol). While on chemotherapy you will be encouraged to avoid sunlight. It is then essential that you have a vitamin D supplement, and if you are not a vegetarian, I recommend D3. Fresh air is good for the body, mind, and soul, and although you should be cautious of sun exposure, it is good to get fresh air on a covered patio or in a shady spot. In a healthy individual, fifteen minutes a day in sunlight is enough to give you the daily quota.

Vitamin D is also found in certain animal fats. Given low-fat diets and the threat of skin cancer from sun exposure, we tend to avoid animal fat and sunshine. Vitamin D is essential to building our immune system and strengthening our bones. In fact, in most cancer diagnoses, the individuals always have a deficiency of Vitamin D (Cowan, 2004). Bone marrow creates our blood cells, and the chemotherapy attacks this area. Fortifying your bone marrow is necessary to keep your blood cells producing while on chemotherapy. Vitamin D is also essential for proper utilization of calcium which is another factor necessary for bone health (Ottoboni & Ottoboni, 2002).

Vitamin B

This vitamin is essential to counteract the stress hormone cortisol. This is really important as anyone diagnosed with cancer has high stress levels. The change in lifestyle, new treatment regime, facing mortality, and feeling terrible or in pain cannot be set aside. The clearer we can focus, the better to adjust to this 'new normal' and concentrate on quality of life. In taking Vitamin B, make sure you stay within guidelines. Don't mega-dose. Although low toxic capability, an imbalance in the diet can cause problems. In particular, Niacin, B3, can cause temporary flushing of the skin (heat sensation).

B vitamin is water-soluble meaning it will not store in the body. When Vitamin B is excreted the urine is a bright chartreuse colour. Since the body expels excess Vitamin B, it needs to be a daily supplement.

Vitamin C

Vitamin C is essential for immunity and nutrition, but it is critical for attacking cancer cells. Vitamin C is important in cancer destruction since extreme stress uses up huge amounts of this vitamin. Vitamin C is an antiviral substance that helps form the collagen (glue) between healthy cells, which prevent viruses from piercing the cell walls. Viruses can multiply only after they have entered a cell (Mindell & Hopkins, 2003). Vitamin C works to neutralize free radicals. Cancer cannot exist or grow in an oxygen-rich and slightly alkaline (pH 7.36) environment (Coldwell, 2017). Cancer cells pull carbohydrates to them for easier energy metabolism. In other words, cancer loves sugar. Vitamin C gives the 'appearance' of a carbohydrate to cancer cells. The cells absorb the vitamin C quickly; however, in a cancer cell (nonaerobic environment), this vitamin converts to hydrogen peroxide and it attacks from the inside out. Unfortunately, we cannot eat enough vitamin C to fight the cancer. Orally, vitamin C is weaker but effective; however, in an IV it can increase hydrogen peroxide levels deep in the tissue where cancer cells live. Some sources claim that IV therapy with vitamin C poses good options; however, the research about this is not solid at the time of this book's publication.

Vitamin C is an antioxidant as described earlier and can pass through the blood brain barrier. The more Vitamin C in the brain cells, the less likely chemicals can penetrate the barrier. You may recall that one of the side effects of prolonged chemotherapy is 'brain fog' which is the chemicals attaching to the brain cells. Therefore, vitamin C protects the brain (Blaylock, 1994). A side effect of too much vitamin C is a minor laxative effect.

Folic acid

Folic acid helps your body produce and maintain new cells and build red blood cells. Folic acid can be found in dark green leafy products such as kale, spinach, and romaine lettuce. Some chemotherapy drugs such as methotrexate may block folic acid production (Mindell & Hopkins, 2003). In addition, people with low levels of folic acid are more prone to depression (Frei, Quillin, & Bloomfield, 1996). With the stress of cancer, reducing any risk of depression is essential.

❖ Other natural information

Bentonite

Bentonite clay has antibacterial and anti-inflammatory properties. This clay can be taken orally or applied to the skin as a paste mixed with water. Bentonite has the ability to bond with unwanted substances (toxins) in the digestive tract by adsorbent action (Pathak, 2020).

Once the chemotherapy session is over, it is important to get the chemo out of the body as soon as possible so healing can occur. Taking bentonite (human grade - liquid or capsule) helps to do this. I provided my husband with bentonite capsules for three days every morning and evening from the day of treatment. Also, for sores that are slow to heal, add a paste of bentonite and water and then air dry, or better yet, use aloe vera gel instead of water. It is very benign and does not cause discomfort. Leave the paste on and only wash once daily, reapply as necessary.

Oxygen/alkaline environment

Noble Prize Winner Otto Warburg scientifically proved that cancer cells cannot grow or exist in an oxygen rich environment. Nobel Prize Winner Max Plant proved that cancer cannot grow in an alkaline environment. So, it is well recognized that the way to stop cancer is by creating oxygen, alkaline cellular environments (Coldwell, 2017). In order to change a body from acidic to alkaline, you must eliminate refined sugar because cancer cells love sugar. Eat lots of fruits and vegetables. Fresh lemonade has the ability to help change your body to alkaline (see recipe below). Maintain your body's pH levels between 7.1 and 7.3 in the blood and 7.36 in the body (measured by saliva or urine). To do this you can purchase pH sticks that guide you through the process where you either spit on the stick or pee in a cup (see section titled "Where can I buy these herbs and vitamins?").

Lemonade recipe

> Squeeze the juice out of a lemon. Add 2 tablespoons of authentic pure maple syrup or the amount that suits your taste. Add 10 to 12 ounces of water. Add a small amount of ground cayenne pepper. Stir. Gradually increase the amount of cayenne to half a teaspoon. Drink this three times per day minimum (Coldwell, 2017).
>
> Note: Lemon is a strong anti-carcinogen. It has a powerful effect on cysts and tumours. Cayenne has capsaicin which potentially reduces cancer cell growth.

CBD oil

I would be remiss if I did not mention CBD oil. CBD products are cannabis-based, but because they contain little to no THC, they don't get you high. When I was studying traditional natural health, CBD oil was deemed illegal so I didn't know all the healing properties that it offered. Upon legalization in Canada, my husband was able to try it. The effect was dramatic in that he had more energy, more restful sleeps, and fewer bad days between treatments. To determine the concentration right for you, here is a guideline: https://cbd-oil-canada.ca/cbd-oil-dosage/.

There are also medical cannabis clinics that you should consult which will help point you to the right product and in some cases provide coverage through benefits.

Neuropathy

Another disturbing side effect with some chemotherapy is neuropathy – a numbness and tingling in hands and feet. With time this can remove all sensation in the lower legs, feet, and hands. Cold exposure is very painful. I was hesitant to add this to the book, as my husband experienced neuropathy and I wondered if what we were doing was working. In speaking with his oncologist, he explained that he was so impressed that my husband's neuropathy had not gotten worse and in fact had resided somewhat. He had never seen that. So, with this confirmation, let me tell you what we did. My husband does have numbness and tingling; however, he has never lost feeling after two years on this type of chemo. We utilized an herbal blend designed for diabetic neuropathy. This blend is called Nerve Miracle. Just to reiterate, the neuropathy still happened, but it didn't get worse, and after time it is less, even with continued chemotherapy. So this is one of these longer-term results. For my husband this was critical since he plays guitar and did not want to lose that ability. Remember the things that are important in maintaining our quality of life. See the next section for where you can buy this blend. Another small point to add – refrain from touching cold, use gloves. My husband was careful not to drink cold beverages as this affected his throat, felt like he was losing his voice.

Where Can I Buy These Herbs and Vitamins?

I truly dislike when I read about something and the only way I can find it is if I purchase it directly from the author or company writing the book. My intent here is to make this very simple and cost-effective. You have enough to deal with. There are other options of where to purchase these herbs and vitamins, but for the purpose of this book and convenience, these are retailers where I know the product is effective and of good quality. If you purchase elsewhere and do not feel like the product is doing anything for you, remember 'buyer beware' and try another brand to ensure it is not a quality issue. There are a lot of companies out there selling herbs and vitamins that are packed with fillers rather than concentrated elements. CTV News reported on John Nolan, Founder & Director of the Nutritional Research Center, Ireland. His research confirmed that 63% of Canadian herbal supplements tested lacked the nutritional value stated on the label. Health Canada guidelines for Natural Health Products require that the quantity of medicinal ingredients be a minimum of 80 per cent of the label claim. Dr. Nolan explained that by allowing 80%, some companies work towards the lower limits of herb content hence, increasing profit by adding non value added fillers. The reality is Health Canada should expect products contain 100% of the label claim or people cannot expect to see a benefit from the natural health product (Jones, 2021). You can watch the interview here https://www.ctvnews.ca/health/many-supplements-for-vision-loss-do-not-achieve-their-label-claim-researcher-says-1.5468929.

Marigold and lemon balm are very easy to grow, and in the springtime, they can be found in most greenhouses. However, if they are out of season or you don't have the time or place to grow these plants, you can buy them in teabag form. Follow the directions in this book.

Herbaria teas – Traditionally Wild-Crafted and Cultivated Herbal Teas Since 1949

http://herbarianorthamerica.com/

For all remaining herbs, vitamins, and pH sticks, I recommend *Swanson Vitamins*. These products are of good quality and the prices are very reasonable. I will provide the direct link, but note if you need something urgently you can purchase Swanson products on Amazon. However the prices here are more expensive.

Think about your ability to swallow pills before you purchase. Many of these products come in liquid form but also in tablets (hard surface, various shapes) or in gel capsule (cylinder shape but different volumes). When you find the product you are looking for, you can see what form it comes in.

Swanson Vitamins

www.swansonvitamins.com

For neuropathy this is the only product where we found results. It is a USA purchase.

Nerve Miracle – Diabetes Doctor www.diabetesdoctor.com

The recipe for Chemo Ease

I have listed quite a few products and I don't want this to be overwhelming. Here is how you can make your own blend of Chemo Ease to reduce the volume of things to take.

Purchase the liquid version, no alcohol, with the same volume of each product (i.e. 1 ounce):

- Astragalus
- Horsetail
- Ginkgo biloba
- Milk thistle
- Burdock
- Red clover

Pour each bottle into a jar/bottle that holds at least 6 ounces and mix. Store in cupboard (not in direct light).

Pour 1 teaspoon into some water or juice twice daily – once in the morning, and once in the evening. Six ounces of liquid will provide you with enough Chemo Ease for 18 days.

I also purchase liquid vitamin D3 and add it to the morning drink.

What Else Can You Do?

You need to take control of your care and be informed. One of the easiest ways to monitor your progress is to keep records of your blood work. Prior to chemotherapy, the oncologist will have your blood work analyzed to ensure you have enough cell consistency to handle the chemotherapy. Ask for a copy of this report. It is your personal information, and it is not uncommon to have a copy. You should do this for all medical testing and assessments so you have a comprehensive file readily available.

I don't expect you to understand all of it, but there are some simple things you can monitor.

Go over your blood work report with your healthcare practitioner. Ask them how you can increase any low values whether it be through taking a supplement or eating a type of food. Reference this book for guidance and to help with your problem-solving. In my husband's case, he was taking chemotherapy every two weeks which started with blood work. We were able to see quickly any changes and problem-solve how to increase a deficit or if our previous solution was working.

My husband had a PICC line (IV line inserted) and we found that after chemo, and again after having his dressing changed where they flush the line, he was very tired and listless with memory fog, chills, and muscle pain. We found that the number of flushes was overhydrating him (too much water in the system when given by IV). This isn't a problem for the majority, but in his case, it was really affecting him. Under the oncologist's guidance, the volume of flushing was safely reduced and it made a significant difference for him. We were also told that sometimes in the case of dressing changes, the flush, if administered too quickly (pushed in by syringe), can also affect the way the person feels afterwards.

I don't know if my husband was just sensitive to medication, but we also found that the concentration of steroids given to him at the time of chemotherapy made him extremely hyper, agitated, and oversensitive. After speaking with the oncologist, this concentration was reduced. I emphasize this again about how critical it is to have these frank discussions with your healthcare team. There are solutions, but if you don't explain or ask, you will never get another option.

It is critical that a person undergoing treatment gets proper sleep to heal. When on chemotherapy, the treatment includes steroids which can make it very difficult to sleep. We have tried different herbal combinations, but quite frankly I found that when in the process of treatment (the day of treatment and after treatment if you carry a bottle), the drugs are too strong and herbs do not work. Talk to your oncologist for a solution for this day or these three days.

On another note – taking medication for other ailments while on chemotherapy may result in a different effect. Note that your blood levels are low so the medicine can absorb into the tissue faster and may cause side effects that you did not experience before. It is critical that you monitor how you feel and discuss any differences with your doctor. Never stop a medication 'cold turkey' as many pharmaceuticals will cause other problems. Some medications you need to reduce over time. It took us a few tries with blood thinners to find the right brand and dosage to stop side effects for my husband and eventually move to herbs.

Again, I cannot say this enough: you need to keep a log and explain as best as you can how you feel and when. Don't assume that feeling awful is all attributed to chemotherapy and that there is nothing else that can be done. It is up to you to question and understand options.

Another critical piece of information that was recommended to us is when your CT scan comes back with no significant growth or shrinkage, take a chemotherapy session off. So, within a three-month period between CT scans and chemo every two weeks, my husband will take one session off when he has no significant growth. This provides time for his body to heal. We would time this with holidays or life events, for example. I believe that in getting so concerned with fighting the disease, we keep pushing and don't think about taking a rest for body and soul. Think of your rest as a reward for no significant growth!! Again, your oncologist will be able to advise you for your personal schedule.

Conclusion

In conclusion, what can I say...I wish you the very best in maintaining your quality of life for as long as you have. I truly hope that this book has provided you with some glimmer of information that helps you feel better. Remember, it is quality not quantity, comfort over fight, and appreciation for good days in your 'new normal' life. Make and relive good memories, have good belly laughs, and kick yours shoes off, put your feet on the grass and just breathe.

My wish for you is to create and to share moments by problem-solving and questioning how you can feel better in the time you have left.

References

Blaylock, R. L. (1994). *Excitotoxins: The taste that kills.* Health Press.

Canadian Cancer Society. (2021). www.cancer.ca

CBD Oil Canada. (2021). https://cbd-oil-canada.ca/cbd-oil-dosage/

Coldwell, L. (2017). *The only cancer patient cure.* 21st Century Press.

Cowan, T. S. (2004). *The fourfold path to healing.* New Trends Publishing.

Fitzgerald, P. (2001). *The detox solution.* Illumination Press.

Frei, B., Quillin, P., & Bloomfield, H. (1996). *Preventions, healing with vitamins.* Rodale Press, Inc.

Illich, I. (1994). *Brave New Biocracy: Healthcare from Womb to Tomb.* New Perspectives Quarterly, Winter94, Vol. 11, Issue 1.

Jones, A. M. (2021.) *Many supplements for vision loss do not achieve their label claim, researcher says.* https://www.ctvnews.ca/health/many-supplements-for-vision-loss-do-not-achieve-their-label-claim-researcher-says-1.5468929

Mindell, E., & Hopkins, V. (2003). *Prescription alternatives.* Bottom Line Books.

Mowrey, D. (1993). *Herbal tonic therapies.* Keats Publishing.

Ottoboni, F., & Ottoboni, A. (2004). *The modern nutritional diseases.* Vincente Books Inc.

Pathak, N. (2020). *Health benefits of bentonite.* www.WebMD.com

Snyder, B. (2021, April 15). *Top spenders in big pharma.* Fierce Pharma. www.fiercepharma.com

Wilson-Hare, L. (2007). *Surviving stress: A study of professional women's stress levels, their genetic resiliency, and herbal adaptogens as an effective intervention.* Universal Publishers. https://www.universal-publishers.com/book.php?method=ISBN&book=1581123647

Lightning Source UK Ltd.
Milton Keynes UK
UKHW020817031121
393263UK00007B/266